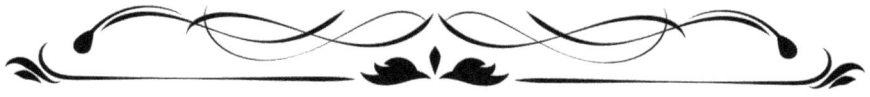

IDENTIFYING CHILDHOOD TRAUMA *and* IMPROVING *Trauma-informed Care* *in* BEHAVIORAL HEALTH

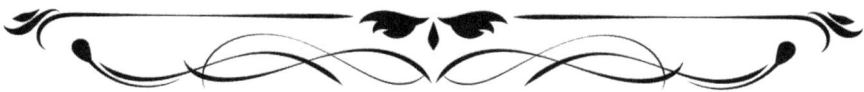

A Systematic Investigation

DR. H. MINOR, DNP

Imperium Publishing
1097 N. 400th Rd
Baldwin City, KS, 66006

www.imperiumpublishing.com

Acknowledgments

AFTER YEARS OF HARD work, time, and effort, I would like to acknowledge those that supported me along the way. This includes the faculty and advisors at Maryville University, the preceptors who were willing to share their time and knowledge with me, the hospital and staff that welcomed my research, and my friends and family.

Dedication

I WANT TO DEDICATE this work to my supportive and loving husband, Jason, and my wonderful children. If it were not for their love and support, I would not have been able to accomplish this. They were the ones that supported me through exhaustion, stress, and many tears. They lifted me when I thought I could go no further. They held me when I failed and celebrated with me when I succeeded. Most importantly, they never let me quit.

Jason, Jayden, Saphira, Serenity, and Scarlett, there will never be words to express how much I love you, but I will spend my last breath trying.

Table of Contents

LIST OF FIGURES...x
LIST OF TABLES xi
ABSTRACT..xiii
Chapter 1 INTRODUCTION 15
    Problem 15
    Purpose 16
    Background Knowledge 16
    Type of Inquiry 17
    Background..17
    Significance 19
        Significance to Nursing Practice 20
        Significance to Advanced Practice Nursing Practice 22
        Significance to Healthcare 23
    Project Support 24
    Benefits of Project to Practice 24
Chapter 2 LITERATURE SYNTHESIS 27
    Search History..27
    Integrated Review of Literature 28

Effect of Childhood Trauma on Adults............................28

Providing Trauma-informed Care...................................30

Childhood Trauma Questionnaire................................32

Literature Critique 34

Strengths of Evidence..34

Weaknesses of Evidence...36

Gaps...37

Limitations..38

Concepts and Definiti0ns..38

Theoretical Framework..39

Chapter 3 METHODOLOGY 43

Design..44

Inclusion Criteria 45

Exclusion Criteria...46

Data Collection Instrument 47

Validity and Reliability 47

Analysis Plan 47

Budget 48

Timeline 49

Protection of Human Subjects.......................................49

Chapter 4 FINDINGS 51

Methods of Evaluation 51

Quantitative (or Qualitative) methods 52

Setting..52

Sample 53

Structure of Intervention 53

Data Quality and Adequacy 54

Ethical Considerations 54

Conflict of Interest 55

Data Analysis and Presentation of Data 55

Descriptive Statistics 56

Variability...56
Results 57
    Outcomes of Intervention 57
    Facilitators and Barriers 60
    Unintended Consequences 61
Chapter 5 DISCUSSION 65
    Strengths 66
    Limitations 67
        Missing Data 68
        Post-Implementation Insights 69
    Interpretation 69
    Implications for Future Research 70
    Implications for Practice 71
    Implications for Healthcare policy 71
    Recommendations and Conclusions 71
        Plan for Sustainability 72
        Plan for Dissemination...73
    REFERENCES 75

LIST OF FIGURES

Figure 1. *Identification of Childhood Trauma* 59

Figure 2. *Communication of Trauma History*..............................59

Figure 2. *Adults with Trauma* 62

LIST OF TABLES

Table 1. *Budget Plan*..48
Table 2. *Identification of Childhood Trauma* 59
Table 3. *Communication of Trauma History* 59

Abstract

Purpose: To improve Trauma-informed care by improving the identification and communication of childhood trauma.

Background: Childhood trauma can affect people throughout their lifespan. The Childhood Trauma Questionnaire (CTQ) is a reliable and valid tool to identify childhood trauma. Trauma identification and communicating among caregivers is an important part of Trauma-informed care. Trauma-informed care has been shown to be an effective way to care for patients who have experienced trauma in their lives.

Methods: This was done by training nurses on Trauma-informed care, the CTQ, and the importance of communication of a patient's trauma history. The nurses were responsible for providing the CTQ to the patients to fill out in the privacy of their rooms. The CTQs were then collected and scored, and the results were reported to the communication log that the staff utilized.

Results: Trauma history was inquired about in 223 patients out of the 225 pre-intervention (95%). Post-intervention only 86 patients out of 139 completed the CTQ (62%). Pre-intervention 21 patients, out of the 86 that trauma was identified in had their trauma history communicated (24%). Post-intervention trauma history was communicated on 61 out of 62 patients (98%). Pre-intervention, 36.6% of patients reported having a trauma history. Post-intervention, 53.06% reported having trauma.

Conclusions: The CTQ was used less frequently than the previous methods of identifying trauma. However, trauma was identified more frequently. The communication of identified trauma increased substantially.

ONE:

Introduction

CHILDHOOD TRAUMA HAS BEEN linked to significant mental health issues for adults (Heany et al., 2017). Nearly two-thirds of all children experience trauma by 16 years of age (Substance Abuse and Mental Health Services Association [SAMHSA], 2022). The high number of people facing traumatic experiences throughout their lives makes it imperative that trauma is identified and addressed by healthcare providers.

Problem

Healthcare staff in the Behavioral Health Unit (BHU) at the identified hospital have received education on providing Trauma-informed care. However, patients with childhood trauma are not receiving Trauma-informed care. There is concern regarding trauma being identified well and communicated amongst staff. Trauma-informed care cannot be clinically delivered if trauma is not recognized, and it is not communicated to the people providing the care.

The practice proposed for the Doctor of Nursing Practice (DNP) scholarly project was the utilization of the Childhood Trauma Questionnaire (CTQ), which will improve the identification of childhood trauma. This information was used to improve staff communication of the questionnaire results, which allowed for improvement in overall Trauma-informed care. By doing so, staff are better equipped to provide interventions to address previous trauma, specifically as part of overall Trauma-informed care. Increasing awareness of childhood trauma allows the staff to provide the Trauma-informed care that they have already been trained to provide.

Purpose

The purpose of the scholarly project was to improve the delivery of Trauma-informed care at the BHU. Thus, the aim was to improve the ability of healthcare staff to provide Trauma-informed care. A secondary aim of this project was to improve the identification of childhood trauma utilizing the CTQ. Another secondary aim was to improve communication among healthcare workers when someone has a history of trauma.

Background Knowledge

The author has been practicing as a Registered Nurse (RN) for 17 years, at the bedside and in various leadership positions throughout the hospital and mental health environments. This scholar's firsthand knowledge has provided the experience to undertake this project. Holding a master's degree in nursing (MSN) and working towards a Doctor of Nursing practice (DNP) also provided significant education and knowledge to be applied throughout the project. As a DNP prospect, this scholar specialized as a Psychiatric Mental Health Nurse Practitioner (PMHNP). Therefore, the education received was focused on mental health. As a soon to be PMHNP, this researcher wanted to address this deficiency in the care provided at the designated hospital.

Type of Inquiry

This project was a practice improvement project, directly addressing the identification of patient trauma history and its communication of it amongst health care workers, assisting them in providing effective and sensitive care. This project could influence the patient's experience of their care, which could lead to future improvements in care. Due to the successful completion and positive outcomes from this project, it will likely lead to policy revision and hospital-wide implementation.

Outcomes assessed for this project included training staff, the frequency of administration of the CTQ, and the improvement of communication of patient trauma history. Training staff was measured by the training sign-in sheet. The administration of the CTQ was measured using a chart review. Improvement of communication was measured by audit. The key to the successful implementation of this project was education and frequent rounding and observation with the nursing staff.

Background

Screening for trauma, including childhood trauma, is a component of Trauma-informed care. Trauma-informed care is a way of approaching the care provided to people that allows for transparency and sensitivity to what each individual person has been through in their lives and how those experiences may be connected to their current situation.

Nursing is the largest profession in healthcare, according to Wakefield et al. (2021); a profession that is highly unutilized in driving change. With nurses providing direct patient care, they are a resource that can be used to improve patient care through trauma identification and providing Trauma-informed care. However, nurses need to be given the resources to accomplish this task.

Childhood trauma is related to many adult mental health issues. Behr Gomes Jardim et al. (2018) performed a cross-sectional study to determine the influence of childhood abuse and trauma on depression and suicide risk later in life. They found that childhood neglect, as well as abuse, was a significant precursor to suicide risk. Oquendo et al. (2020) also determined that childhood trauma was a predictor for suicidal ideation variability and that it caused a greater increase in suicidal ideation after being exposed to a stressor.

Gaweda et al. (2019) performed a study to determine the relationship between childhood trauma, psychotic-like experiences (PLE), and depression on suicidal ideation. They found a five-fold increase in suicidal ideation for those who suffered from childhood trauma and PLEs and a six-fold increase in those with depression. Angelakis et al. (2019) found a two to three-fold increase in suicide attempts in adults when there was a history of childhood trauma. In addition, Grattan et al. (2019) found that trauma history is associated with not only suicidal ideation but also non-suicidal self-injurious behavior and aggression.

Identifying trauma history is the first step in Trauma-informed care. As stated previously, Trauma-informed care is a way of approaching the care provided to people that allows for transparency and sensitivity to what each individual person has been through in their lives and how those experiences may be connected to their current situation. Trauma-informed care has been shown to significantly improve patient satisfaction as well as increase planned discharges, as opposed to people leaving against medical advice (AMA) (Hales et al., 2018).

Bloomfield et al. (2020) performed a systematic review to determine effective treatment in patients who have a traumatic past. They found that actions such as acceptance, emotional regulation, and other aspects of Trauma-informed care have proven quite effective.

Ranjbar et al. (2020) explained that providing Trauma-informed care will allow for the mental health population to be served more effectively. They go on to explain that this holistic approach helps to improve the lives of both the provider and the patients.

The research supports the identification of trauma history and providing Trauma-informed care to patients. However, the question remains: how can that be accomplished? Herein lies some barriers to addressing these issues. There are many ways that trauma can be identified. One could simply ask about trauma history or perform a screening tool. However, these can illicit such feelings as embarrassment and fear for the patient, as well as the withholding of information. Another barrier is that there is no standardization or requirement on how to identify trauma history. The solution is selecting one tool to identify trauma history and use it on every patient.

The CTQ is a self-administered questionnaire that is utilized to identify a history of childhood trauma. The patient is provided with the questionnaire and instructed to complete it themselves, allowing for privacy and reflection. Xiang et al. (2021) found that the CTQ was a reliable questionnaire in assessing previous trauma. They also found that it did not matter how long since the trauma had occurred or whether the patient was experiencing any issues now or not. Georgieva et al. (2021) did a systematic review and found that the results of the CTQ were consistent and able to be replicated. They stated that this showed the quality of the instrument.

Significance

Implementing this project, enabled the nursing staff, Advanced Practice Providers (APNs), and physicians to provide Trauma-informed care. Being informed of a trauma history allows all these specialties to be sensitive to the individual needs of each patient. This scholarly project also directly affected communication amongst staff, allowing for improved quality of care.

Nursing

Often, a patient's first interaction with medical staff is with a nursing professional conducting an assessment by gathering information about the patient's physiological, psychological, environmental status, and history. This initial assessment informs the diagnosis and care for the patient. This initial assessment is often the introduction of the patient to the provider and can, therefore, be susceptible to anchoring bias. Fully inclusive nursing assessment provide greater context for diagnosis and decisions concerning treatment and care (Dalton et al., 2018). Therefore, a screening tool that provides greater insight into a patient's psychological condition is beneficial for nurses in their initial assessments of patients.

Assessment of patients with mental and behavioral health concerns or disorders can pose a challenge due to the complexities and externalities associated with such disorders. While some externalities may be easily verifiable, such as the use of prescription or illicit drugs through laboratory testing, identifying underlying psychological issues caused by current or past trauma can be more challenging. By immediately understanding that a patient may have had significant trauma by utilizing a screening tool, nurses are empowered to utilize Trauma-informed care training to deliver better care to the patient early. Dalton et al. (2018) also explored that being resourced with training and knowledge of conditions, nurses may find less frustration in caring for the patient and have greater confidence in their decisions.

Early identification of the need for and the implementation of Trauma-informed care will enable nurses and providers to provide better individualistic care earlier. Additionally, a standardized screening tool provides a baseline for predictive communication between medical providers. This early identification can inform better initial diagnosis and shape the type of care a patient receives prior to a treatment plan being finalized. The early implementation of Trauma-informed care may also increase trust between the patient and providers, thus increasing patient compliance with treatment plans and improving overall patient outcomes.

Empiric Knowing

Empiric knowing is one of five patterns of knowing. Kramer and Chinn (2013) explained that this pattern of knowing focuses on objective facts of nursing. It also involves using theories to test ideas and hypotheses. This project utilized the empiric pattern of knowing by utilizing the objective research presented previously to assist in improving the Trauma-informed care provided on the BHU at the designated hospital.

Ethical Knowing

Kramer and Chinn also explained that ethical knowing, another pattern, focuses on nursing ethics. With ethical knowing one must question if what is being done is responsible and ethical. This project considered ethical knowing by performing the research ethically. No protected health information was utilized in this project. This project was also undertaken with the goal of improving practice, and the care provided to patients.

Emancipatory Knowing

Emancipatory knowing is similar to ethical knowing, only on a larger scale. For this pattern of knowing, according to Kramer and Chinn, one must recognize the inequalities on a societal, cultural, and political level and work to improve these. This scholarly project worked to improve communication and Trauma-informed care surrounding a vulnerable population, those who suffer from mental health and substance use disorders.

Personal Knowing

Kramer and Chinn continued exploring the patterns of knowing, by describing personal knowing. Personal knowing is about focusing inwards. One must identify their one values, strengths, and weaknesses. It is critical for nurses to identify their own potential biases and address those. The focus of this scholarly project was on enabling nurses to improve their communication and to provide Trauma-informed care better. Part of Trauma-informed care is being sensitive to a patient's history and current situation, even if it differs from your own or your beliefs and values.

Aesthetic Knowing

The last pattern of knowing is aesthetic knowing. According to Kramer and Chinn, this pattern of knowing is important for reflection and identifying issues. This pattern allows the nurse to see something that needs done and then accomplish it. The scholarly project addressed this power of knowing directly, by working to fulfill a need. Trauma-identification and improved communication are needed. The issue is the lack of Trauma-informed care due to not adequately identifying patient trauma.

Advanced Practice Nursing

As with the intake assessments that nurses conduct, diagnosis of patients with mental and behavioral health disorders can pose a challenge due to the complexities and externalities associated with such disorders. The childhood trauma screening tool provides additional contextual data points for diagnostic consideration and the development of a treatment plan. As evidenced previously, childhood trauma manifestations can be varied in typology and magnitude and may be an underlying or contributing cause to a disorder. Providers can provide better diagnosis and treatment plans if they are addressing a root cause.

As with nurses, first impressions matter in establishing rapport with the patient. By understanding not only the current psychological state of the patient, but also some of the factors that have led to that state, practitioners can employ methods of interaction with the patient that are best suited for their needs. The patient will likely see the provider as more empathetic and trustworthy. This can lead to better rapport with the patient. Ultimately, trust can be improved by improving the patient's understanding and adjusting approaches accordingly.

Healthcare

The marginal cost of implementing an early childhood trauma screening tool within a national healthcare system is negligible as it only consumes a few minutes of time from a healthcare provider and the patient. The negligible cost association makes any beneficial increase in patient outcome or quality of care cost-effective. Further, improved quality of care that leads to better patient outcomes would likely generate a net cost savings from a decrease in patients leaving against medical advice, resulting in a decrease in subsequent readmissions.

The increase in quality of care may lead to fewer suicides. Suicides have immense societal and economic impacts. The suicide of a loved one is a traumatic event and may increase the total number of psychological trauma-related admissions. From a larger, economic perspective, US Government agencies generally value a life at $11,000,000 utilizing a value of statistical life calculation (Viscusi, 2020). Therefore, if the implementation of a childhood trauma screening tool and improved communication, during the admission process, prevents a single suicide, the economic savings is $11,000,000.

Project Support

The support for this scholarly project has been significant thus far. The BHU Director of Nursing (DON) assisted in developing the project idea. She was able to identify the need to improve the Trauma-informed care that was provided to patients. With that need identified, this scholar presented her with this project propsal. The DON was very supportive of the project from the start. Together, the DON and scholar presented the project proposal to the Physicians and Nurse Practitioners for input. Both specialties expressed their support for the project. All of the professionals mentioned agreed to offer their assistance during the implementation phase of the Scholarly project. A space on the BHU was also identified to hold training and education in.

Benefit of Project to Practice

Despite Trauma-informed care being shown to assist patients during their healthcare treatments, as evidenced previously, the staff on the BHU were not identifying trauma. The BHU is designated to provide care to inpatients going through substance detoxification, as well as those suffering from mental health issues. These afflictions have been shown to have a direct relation with previous trauma. However, the staff had not been enabled to provide Trauma-informed care, due to lack of identification of trauma. This scholarly project allowed the staff to be aware of trauma history so that they could provide the Trauma-informed care that is appropriate for each patient on their individual roads to recovery.

Conclusion

Most adults have a history of childhood trauma, as evidenced previously. This has been shown to have the potential to affect them in many ways negatively. Specifically, childhood trauma has been linked to depression and suicidal ideation. Healthcare providers practicing Trauma-informed care have been shown to impact these patients' outcomes positively.

The goal of the scholarly project was to improve the delivery of Trauma-informed care, which the nurses have been trained to provide. This was achieved by first identifying childhood trauma, utilizing the CTQ, and then requiring this to be communicated amongst the team in specific ways. This enabled the providers to deliver the care they have been trained to provide.

As the largest profession in healthcare, nursing has the ability to drive change. Nurses are a largely untapped resource. This practice and quality improvement project capitalized on that resource by enabling them to provide effective and patient-sensitive care in a way that is most appropriate for each individual patient.

TWO:

Literature Synthesis

THE POPULATION THAT WAS targeted is adult patients who are admitted to the BHU. These patients are admitted with acute substance use or are experiencing a mental health crisis. The intervention was performing the CTQ on the admission of patients to this unit and then communicating the results. The CTQ is a screening form that the patient can fill out privately. It will help to identify trauma history.

Search History

A search was performed based on the research question stated previously. The databases searched were: Complementary Index, CINAHL, SocINDEX, Medline Complete, JSTOR Journals, and Academic Search Complete. The following Boolean Phrases were utilized in the search: Childhood Trauma Questionnaire AND Trauma-informed care, CTQ AND childhood trauma, CTQ AND childhood trauma AND adult psych, trauma history OR childhood trauma AND Trauma-informed care, childhood trauma AND adult psych, Childhood trauma AND adult depression, trauma history AND adult psych.

The results were then filtered using the following parameters: 2018 to present, English language, peer-reviewed, full-text. Of the resulting articles, 30 were initially selected based on a review of their abstracts. This number was reduced to 16 after a full critical review of each article, selecting only the primary research articles that most closely fit the question at hand.

Integrated Review of Literature

To address the research question, one must understand three things. First, the profound effect that childhood trauma has on a person throughout their life. Second, the importance and effectiveness of providing Trauma-informed care. Third, the data supporting the use of the CTQ.

Effect of Childhood Trauma on Adults

Trauma has a significant impact on people. This impact is not just immediate, or shortly thereafter, but throughout their life (Behr Gomes Jardim et al., 2018; Cay et al., 2022; Cilia Vincenti et al., 2021; Copeland et al., 2018; Gaweda et al., 2019; Grattan et al., 2019; Hales et al., 2018; Isobel et al., 2020; Kratzer et al., 2021; Oquendo et al., 2020; Ozakar Akca et al., 2021). It is well-accepted that trauma history is related to the current state of someone's mental health (Hales et al., 2018; Isobel et al., 2020; Kratzer et al., 2021); however, the effects of trauma on the human psyche are vast and continue to be studied.

Trauma has been linked to many issues, both mental and physical (Kratzer et al., 2021). Some of the lasting effects that childhood trauma has on people will be demonstrated in this section. Childhood trauma showed positive correlations with symptoms of pain, post-traumatic stress disorder (PTSD), dissociation, and concentration (Kratzer et al., 2021; Oquendo et al., 2020). In addition, cumulative childhood trauma exposure has also been found to be associated with numerous adult psychiatric disorders, such as Schizophrenia and Bipolar Disorder (Cay et al., 2022; Gaweda et al., 2019; Kratzer et al., 2021), as well as lower self-esteem (Ozakar Akca et al., 2021). Trauma history plays a huge role in the psyche of people for years to come.

These challenges could also contribute to day-to-day issues. For example, functionality issues such as failure to hold a steady job or maintain relationships are also contributed to childhood trauma (Copeland et al., 2018). Cumulative episodes of childhood trauma increase the risk of these functionality issues (Copeland et al., 2018). Trauma has life-long effects and needs to be considered in the treatment of patients.

Childhood trauma has a significant impact on adult behaviors as well. For example, childhood trauma, specifically physical abuse, appears to lead to aggression and impulsivity in adults (Grattan et al., 2019; Oquendo et al., 2020). Aggression and impulsivity, in turn, have been found to predict suicidal behavior (Grattan et al., 2019). This may be due to a link between those behaviors and depression.

Childhood trauma is linked to depression, suicidal ideation, and non-suicidal self-injury behavior (Gaweda et al., 2019; Grattan et al., 2019; Ozakar Akca et al., 2021). This shows why it is imperative to identify a history of trauma in patients that are being treated. This knowledge could potentially alter their treatment plans or the course of their treatment.

When speaking of suicide risk or suicidal ideation, it is important to consider childhood trauma as a major factor. In multiple studies, past traumatic experiences were associated with an increased probability of suicide in adults (Gaweda et al., 2019; Grattan et al., 2019; Ozakar Akca et al., 2021). Some studies even showed that childhood trauma can go as far as to predict suicide risk as an adult and late in life (Behr Gomes Jardim et al., 2018; Gaweda et al., 2019). Identifying childhood trauma is imperative when treating these patients. If childhood trauma is identified in patients, it can be considered in providing their care and developing their treatment plans.

It was found that childhood maltreatment is a predicts late-life suicide risk, even controlling depression (Behr Gomes Jardim et al., 2018). Due to this, it is important to identify factors for suicide risk besides depression. This shows how important it is to screen all patients for trauma history.

Gaweda et al. (2019) found that childhood trauma and psychotic-like experiences (PLE) were associated with a five-fold increase in suicidal behavior. They also found that depression was associated with a six-fold increase in suicidal behavior. With staggering statistics like that, it is essential that healthcare providers act.

Although childhood trauma is linked to many issues that continue to affect people as adults, there is a surprising lack of understanding among healthcare providers. The lack of understanding comes in many forms. One is that healthcare providers do not always realize how much trauma history is related to current behavior in adults (Cilia Vincenti et al., 2021).

It was also well accepted that trauma history was related to the current state of adult mental health clients, although how it is related differed amongst participants. The lack of agreement among providers is from either not understanding or having differing opinions on how trauma history is related to adult ailments (Isobel et al., 2020). In other words, they know it is related but are unclear how.

Providing Trauma-informed Care

It was found that 30.9% of adolescents were exposed to at least one traumatic event by the age of 16 (Copeland et al., 2018). With an astounding statistic such as this, it stands to reason that healthcare workers should be providing care that takes this past trauma into consideration. Trauma-informed care provides support for using an individualized approach to treat each patient's individual trauma history and symptoms, hence being Trauma-informed in our care (Behr Gomes Jardim et al., 2018; Cilia Vincenti et al., 2021; Gaweda et al., 2019; Grattan et al., 2019; Hales et al., 2018; Korchmaros et al., 2020; Ozaka Akca et al., 2021). Individualized approaches could include risk management programs as well as care planning (Ozakar Akca et al., 2021).

Depression and cognitive bias play a significant role in the relationship between trauma and suicidal behaviors (Gaweda et al., 2019). It is already known that aggression is associated with trauma and increases the risk of suicidal behaviors. Recognizing and implementing trauma care can help limit these behaviors (Grattan et al., 2019). Again, we can see here that providing Trauma-informed care can improve patient outcomes.

Cay et al. (2022) explained that those with schizophrenia and bipolar disorder reported higher rates of childhood trauma than healthy people. Cay et al. were also able to successfully identify trauma history in these patients when they presented to the hospital. This supports providers asking patients about trauma history despite their psychological state. Knowing at the beginning of a patient's treatment that there is a trauma history can allow a provider to tailor individualized care. This is the premise of Trauma-informed care.

Trauma-informed care has been shown to improve patient satisfaction and is an effective way to treat patients with a traumatic past. Providers have also found satisfaction in Trauma-informed care, which greatly improved the patient's experience. Hales et al. (2018) found that Trauma-informed care implementation caused positive changes in each of the five outcomes assessed: Workplace satisfaction, climate, and procedures (improved by moderate to large effect sizes), client satisfaction, and the number of planned discharges (improved significantly).

When initiating a change in how care is provided, it is natural for some resistance to be met. Korchmaros et al. (2020) initiated and tested two different models for Trauma-informed research-supported treatments. Both models of Trauma-informed care were accepted by staff and shown to be feasible. This shows how easily various methods of providing Trauma-informed care can be integrated and accepted into practice.

Staff have shown positivity about utilizing Trauma-informed care after they learn it and start to practice it (Cilia Vincenti et al., 2021; Korchmaros et al., 2020). This is a good improvement considering nurses reported taking patient's behavior personally prior to learning about Trauma-informed care (Cilia Vincenti et al., 2021). Cilia Vincenti et al. also explained that this could be due to it providing heightened awareness to nurses about the impacts of trauma on patients. Therefore, providing Trauma-informed care also has implications for improving staff experience and retention. Cilia Vinecnti et al. went on to explain that staff satisfaction helps improve patient outcomes, therefore, staff experience with Trauma-informed care is directly related to patient experience with it.

Treatment of patients with psychiatric issues was found to be made more difficult by trauma history due to the definition of trauma, and the treatment of it, varying from psychiatrist to psychiatrist (Isobel et al., 2020). This offers support for moving forward with a standardized Trauma-informed care approach, as well as a standardized identification tool, which will be addressed in the next section.

Childhood Trauma Questionnaire

Trauma has been shown to have a lasting impact on people throughout their lifetime. Trauma-informed care has been shown to have a significant effect on both patients and caregivers. Therefore, the identification and communication of positive trauma histories is imperative to the improvement of patient outcomes. A standard tool, like the CTQ, can be used to achieve this (Aloba et al., 2020; Cay et al., 2022; Hagborg et al., 2022; Kratzer et al., 2021; Oquendo et al., 2020; Ozakar Akca et al., 2021; Schmidt et al., 2018; Xiang et al., 2021).

The CTQ has been found to be well-accepted and a reliable instrument for identifying trauma history (Aloba et al., 2020; Hagborg et al., 2022). It could be used in both clinical screening and research on child maltreatment. The CTQ also showed good internal consistency and psychometric properties (Aloba et al., 2020; Cay et al., 2022; Kratzer et al., 2021), as well as good test-retest reliability (Cay et al., 2022). These studies support the CTQ being a good tool to use.

There were no significant differences among ethnic groups when using the CTQ, and it tests well in both male and female adults (Aloba et al., 2020). It was also shown to be valid and reliable for use in adolescents (Hagborg et al., 2022). This provides support for the tool to be used throughout a significant population of people.

Oquendo et al. (2020) found that childhood trauma was a predictor for suicidal ideation variability and caused a greater increase in suicidal ideation after being exposed to a stressor. They were able to determine this by utilizing the CTQ. Oquendo et al. also found that the CTQ related positively to future aggression. This offers further implications of the CTQ as a predictive tool.

The CTQ, used with a schizophrenic population, was found to be reliable over long intervals, regardless of the patient's symptoms or cognition (Xiang et al., 2021). It was also able to successfully identify trauma history in people with Schizophrenia and Bipolar Disorder, as well as healthy people (Cay et al., 2022). This supports providers asking patients about trauma history despite their psychological state.

The research also provides support for using this tool with patients with many different mental health conditions. The CTQ had a positive correlation with scales used to assess symptoms of PTSD, somatic symptoms such as pain, and dissociative experiences (Kratzer et al., 2021). A history of childhood trauma is often present when adults have those issues.

The CTQ is also comparable to, if not more effective than other scales. The CTQ had a positive correlation with the Suicide Probability Scale (SPS) and Rosenberg Self-Esteem Scale (RSES) (Ozakar Akca et al., 2021). Schmidt et al. (2018) found that while the Adverse Childhood Experiences (ACE) and the CTQ were positively related, the CTQ was more apt at identifying trauma history. Schmidt et al. also explained that the ACE showed some under-reporting. This could possibly be because the CTQ provides more opportunities for the patients to identify their trauma, as it is a longer and more in-depth questionnaire.

Literature Critique

With the literature review complete, it is imperative that a critique be done. While there were some similarities and differences noted within the literature, it still provides a basis for the proposed project. The literature supported the plan of utilizing the CTQ to identify the trauma history of patients. However, the quality of the evidence must be reviewed. Some things that will be considered are conflicts of interest, bias, consent, approval, gaps in research, and any limitations.

Strengths of Evidence

According to Polit and Beck (2021), all research studies must be conducted ethically and not have misconduct. It appears that all studies were performed ethically and free of misconduct. All but five articles specifically stated that they obtained Institutional Review Board (IRB) approval before starting their studies, and that they obtained informed consent from the participants. The five that did not specifically state this did not address IRB approval and consent.

In addition, although funding was obtained through various government programs for some of the research, only three had any potential for bias or conflict of interest. Cilia Vincenti et al. (2021) disclosed that the researcher was employed at the hospital where the research was conducted. While not intentional, there is a chance for unintentional bias, and the author did not address any mitigation factors. In the article from Gaweda et al. (2019), one of the researchers worked for the Ministry of Higher Education. Another researcher worked for the Senior Research Fellowship. Again, this could lead to unintentional bias. Finally, Grattan et al. (2019) disclosed that one of their researchers is a founder and scientific advisor for Safari Health.

The setting of the articles varied from study to study, which is seen as a strength. With the variation in setting, it shows the overall effectiveness of the tool and Trauma-informed care. It also helps to paint a general picture of what trauma can do to people, regardless of whether they are in the community, in a hospital, or in a treatment center.

Another strength is that in almost all the studies the sample was randomly selected. This is a strength because it helps to make the findings more credible. For example, Oquendo et al. (2021) used participants that responded to an advertisement or were at the emergency department with suicidal ideation. If everyone was hand selected to participate in each study, it would be difficult to get a good picture of what the general population would be like.

Weaknesses of Evidence

One weakness that was noted in the literature is the overall sample size. While there are no specific rules with sample size, the larger the size, the better. With this literature review, only six of the 16 articles had over 1,000 participants. All the others were quite a bit smaller, most under 100 participants. For example, Isobel et al. (2020) had a sample size of only 13 psychiatrists. Xiang et al. (2021) had a sample size of only 50 patients. When the sample size is that small, it raises the question of whether the findings would be replicated on a larger scale. However, the authors did show that their results were statistically significant.

Another weakness was that many of the studies included had a specific population targeted for their research. For example, Ozakar Acka et al. (2021) specifically studied university students. Kratzer et al. (2021) used participants that had all previously been diagnosed with PTSD. While it is reasonable to expect researchers to focus on a specific population, it does lend a weakness to the results. It raises the question of whether the results could be replicated with other populations. However, the combined variety of research allows for a larger picture.

Finally, another weakness was that a lot of the articles had predominantly female participants. Grattan et al. (2019) was the outlier, with a predominantly male population. While this does not necessarily mean the results vary from male to female, it also does not mean this could be ruled out. It would be beneficial to have more articles that included a predominantly male population.

Another weakness is that there was no way to control turnover in the studies that had healthcare staff as the participants. Korchmaros et al. (2020) performed a study polling staff at three different intervals. Since staff turnover was not controlled for, the number of respondents varied with each interval, as did the respondent itself. In other words, the results could be varied because the people could be different.

Gaps

As referenced previously, one of the weaknesses of the literature review was that most of the study subjects were female. This leads us to the first gap. There needs to be more research with predominantly male participants. This will show whether the results apply to men as well as women, or whether they are specific to women.

Another gap in the research was utilizing Trauma-informed care and the CTQ on adolescents. While two of the studies identified included adolescents (Aloba et al., 2020; Grattan et al., 2019), one was focused on how trauma affected them, and the other was focused on the CTQ. In addition, Grattan et al. (2019) used participants 12-35 years old, so it was not exclusively adolescents. Due to this gap in research, it is difficult to tell if these interventions would be effective and appropriate for adolescents or not.

An additional gap in the current research was how trauma history was identified in the studies that were focused on Trauma-informed care. The entire premise of the current project was to identify childhood trauma with the CTQ so that Trauma-informed care can be performed. The idea was that one cannot be truly "Trauma-informed" if they do not know what the trauma is.

A final gap in the overall research reviewed was that none were specific to veterans. This bears pointing out because veterans make up a substantial part of our community. Veterans also have the potential to suffer from significant trauma. This leads to questions regarding childhood trauma history and its proclivity to cause adult veterans experiencing traumatic situations to struggle more or less than those with no childhood trauma.

Limitations

To build off one of the research gaps, a major limitation noted amongst the articles reviewed that studied the CTQ was that they were all retrospective. None of the studies tested the CTQ for accuracy with children. The age at which the trauma was experienced was also not evaluated.

Another limitation was the sample size. As stated previously, the sample sizes of the studies were generally quite small, with only a handful of studies over 500 participants. This makes it difficult to ascertain whether the results could be duplicated on a larger scale and, therefore, generalized for the entire population.

In most of the studies, participants were from one area of the country which the study took place in, calling into question the ethnic group variation. This supports the limitation of sample size as well. With the smaller sample size and participants all being from one area, it is hard to rationalize whether the interventions could be appropriate for all.

Cay et al. (2022) reported compelling research about bipolar disorder and Schizophrenia, as well as supporting providers asking patients about trauma history despite their psychological state. Unfortunately, with this article, the CTQ data were originally collected for other purposes. Since data was collected for another purpose initially, that means the researchers had to go through it and select what was pertinent to their current study, which could have skewed the results.

Concepts and Definitions

Childhood Trauma: "refers to a scary, dangerous, violent, or life-threatening event that happens to a child" (Northwestern University, 2020, para. 1).

Dissociation: "involve experiencing a disconnection and lack of continuity between thoughts, memories, surroundings, actions and identity" (Mayo Foundation for Medical Education and Research, 2022, para. 1).

Somatic Symptoms: "Somatic symptom disorder is diagnosed when a person has a significant focus on physical symptoms, such as pain, weakness, or shortness of breath, to a level that results in major distress and/or problems functioning" (American Psychiatric Association, 2021, para. 1).

Trauma-informed Care: "acknowledges that health care organizations and care teams need to have a complete picture of a patient's life situation — past and present — in order to provide effective health care services with a healing orientation" (Center for Healthcare Strategy, 2022, para. 1).

Theoretical Framework

The theory chosen that best fits this project was Cathy Caruth's theory of trauma. Caruth (1996) discusses that experiences of trauma stay with people forever. One needs to share these experiences with others to learn how to heal. Her key takeaways are that trauma changes you, trauma experiences are hard to express, and trauma stays with you throughout your life. If those key points are correct, then trauma should be recognized in people, and they should be treated by professionals accordingly. Their interactions should be individualized based on the patients' personal experiences.

Mambrol (2020) explained that in the traditional trauma model from Cathy Caruth, "trauma is viewed as an event that fragments consciousness and prevents direct linguistic representation. The model draws attention to the severity of suffering by suggesting the traumatic experience irrevocably damages the psyche" (para. 13). This theory directly supported the project because the project was about identifying a patient's trauma history so that appropriate and sensitive care can be provided to the patient, assuming that childhood trauma plays a significant role in adult mental health, as it has been shown to.

Patients may need a way to help them express that they have experienced trauma in the past. This can be done utilizing a screening tool, which was the plan. Trauma can have a long-lasting impact on an individual's life, can be difficult to express, and may require individualized treatment based on the patient's experiences. This project focused on identifying patients who have experienced trauma in the past so that appropriate care can be provided to them. Screening tools can be an effective way to identify patients who may have experienced trauma and can help healthcare professionals tailor their interactions and treatments accordingly.

Trauma theory provides an understanding of the effect of traumatic events on a person's life that renders the victim silent and unable to process the experiences. Caruth (1996) indicated that the theory of trauma explained how the experience of trauma changes a particular way of thinking. Mambrol (2018) implied that traumatic experiences might contribute to lifelong struggles with depression, pain, or substance use. However, these experiences have a profound impact on their life. Individuals need to share their experiences to promote healing.

One of the things Caruth (1996) theorizes was that trauma can be difficult to explain or put into words. This is where the CTQ comes in. The CTQ is meant to be given to the patient to fill out privately, in their own time. This allows for early identification of issues that may be too difficult to discuss.

Conclusion

As evidenced here, trauma has a significant impact on people. This impact can last a lifetime. It is important for healthcare providers to identify the trauma history so that they can get a full picture of what may be affecting a patient. By acknowledging and addressing the impact of trauma on patients, healthcare providers can create a more compassionate and supportive environment for their patients.

It is also important to note that Trauma-informed care is becoming increasingly recognized as a necessary approach in healthcare settings, and this project aligns with this approach. Being Trauma-informed validates victims' experiences which helps them cope with sadness and anger and promotes healing. By enabling staff to adequately identify a history of trauma, they are more apt to provide Trauma-informed care.

The CTQ is a proven and reliable tool to identify a history of childhood trauma in patients. With the help of this tool, healthcare staff can provide care that is sensitive to each individual patient's needs. This will allow them to begin to heal.

THREE:

Methodology

THE IMPACT THAT CHILDHOOD trauma can have on a person is not just immediate or shortly thereafter, but throughout their life (Cay et al., 2022; Cilia Vincenti et al., 2021; Isobel et al., 2020; Kratzer et al., 2021; Oquendo et al., 2020; Ozakar Akca et al., 2021). Childhood trauma has been linked to significant mental health issues for adults (Heany et al., 2017). Therefore, identifying and providing care individualized to a patient's trauma history is essential in the treatment of mental health disorders in adults.

Trauma-informed care is a way of approaching the care provided to people that allows for transparency and sensitivity to what each individual person experienced in their lives and how those experiences may be connected to their current situation. Trauma-informed care has been shown to improve patient satisfaction and is an effective way to treat patients with a traumatic past (Bloomfield et al., 2020; Hales et al., 2018). It has also been shown to improve patient satisfaction and increase planned discharges significantly, as opposed to people leaving against medical advice (AMA) (Hales et al., 2018).

Screening for trauma, including childhood trauma, is a component of Trauma-informed care.

The Childhood Trauma Questionnaire (CTQ) is a reliable and consistent tool for assessing childhood trauma (Georgieva et al., 2021; Xiang et al., 2021). However, minimal research has been done on whether the CTQ aids in providing Trauma-informed care. Patients may need a way to help them express that they have experienced trauma in the past. This can be done utilizing a screening tool, such as the CTQ. Therefore, the purpose of this project was to increase the identification of patients' trauma history so that staff can provide Trauma-informed care.

The project was conducted via quantitative analysis. Baseline data was collected before the research intervention and staff education. This was followed by the eight-week project period. After the eight-week project period, data was collected again.

Design

The participants were adult hospital patients who were admitted to the Behavioral Health Unit at the designated hospital, and the nurses who work in the same unit. The researcher gained access as a student by performing the project in the unit, where they were assigned. The researcher was provided with a patient list for each day included in the project by the Director of Nursing in the utilized unit. Patients were given the Childhood Trauma Questionnaire (CTQ) on admission by hospital nurses and asked to fill it out within 24 hours.

When completed, the CTQ was collected and placed in the patient charts by the nurses. Positive scores were written on the nurse's communication sheets for communicating at the all-unit shift huddle at the beginning of each shift and by nurse-to-nurse during the end-of-shift reports.

This research project was conducted by using the following steps:

1. Data was collected, pre-intervention, on the following:
   a. How many patients were asked about childhood trauma at admission in the previous 8 weeks.
   b. How many patients that were identified as having childhood trauma had it listed on the communication sheet in the previous 8 weeks.
2. Nurses were educated about the project and the process.
3. Provided the CTQ to patients who were included and placed the results on the communication log.
4. Assessed compliance with the project and re-educated staff as needed.
5. Data collection, post-intervention, on 2 the different measures listed previously.
   a. How many patients were asked about childhood trauma at admission during the change period.
   b. How many patients with positive results had their childhood trauma listed on the communication sheet during the change period.

Inclusion Criteria

Inclusion criteria for the patients to be given the Childhood Trauma Questionnaire (CTQ) were the following:

1. They must have been over 18 years of age, per the list provided by the unit director.
2. They were a patient admitted to the Behavioral Health Unit during the change period, January 2024 to May 2024, according to the patient list provided by the unit director.
3. They were English-speaking, according to the hospital's electronic health record (EHR).
4. They were alert and oriented to person, place, and time, according to the EHR.

All races and genders were included in this project so there are no specific inclusion criteria for that.

Inclusion criteria for the nurses to be educated and participate in the intervention, were as follows:

1. They must have been employed as a nurse in the Behavioral Health Unit at the identified hospital, per the nurse list provided by the unit director.
2. They must have been employed during the change period, January 2024 to May 2024, per the list provided by the unit director.

All races and genders were included in this project so there are no specific inclusion criteria for that. In addition, they are already English-speaking, as this is a requirement of their job.

Exclusion Criteria

Patients were excluded from the project for the following reasons:

1. They were 17 years of age or younger, per the list provided by the unit director.
2. They were not patients in the Behavioral Health Unit, as found when comparing the patient list with active patients in the EHR.
3. They were non-English speaking, per the EHR.
4. They had an altered level of consciousness, per the EHR, or per staff report that day.

Exclusion criteria for the nurses to be included in the change process are as follows:

1. They had been floated to the unit from elsewhere in the hospital, to assist, and do not work there per the unit director.
2. They were employed by a staffing agency and contracted to work at the designated hospital, per the unit director.

Data Collection Instruments

Multiple instruments were used to measure whether the CTQ was provided to patients, allowing comparison of the previous method to the change intervention. These instruments included the CTQ, and a Microsoft spreadsheet created solely for the purpose of this project.

Validity and Reliability

The CTQ has been shown to be valid and reliable (Aloba et al., 2020; Hagborg et al., 2022). It is a questionnaire that is given to the patient. It asks them multiple questions to which they rate on a frequency scale. All questions are regarding various aspects of childhood trauma. The Microsoft spreadsheet is not associated with any reliability and validity statistics, since it was created as a place for the purpose of this project.

A staff communication log was reviewed to measure whether the identified trauma was communicated amongst staff from shift to shift. The data obtained included whether the information previously collected was written in the log. This was recorded into the same Microsoft spreadsheet created solely for the purpose of this project.

Analysis Plan

For this project, the researcher collected data on the previously discussed areas. The independent variable was the intervention performed. The dependent variables were the changes this had on the measures or variables being studied. These variables were the pre-versus-post data collection in the measurement areas (trauma identification and communication).

The tests performed were the Z-test and the two-proportion Z-Test to analyze the data obtained. This was done utilizing the Statistical Package for the Social Sciences (SPSS) software. A Z-Test was performed for each individual measure.

Budget

This project used multiple resources including the hospital staff, electronic health records (EHR), office supplies, equipment, and computers. The project was performed at the facility, which means the facility and all its resources are included. Another consideration was the gasoline needed for the researcher to travel to and from the project site.

The project took approximately eight weeks to complete, not including the planning that had been done, and the completion of the five-chapter report. The budget for this project was based on anticipated costs for the completion of this project (Table 1). While other costs would typically be incurred, such as office supplies, computers, the internet, and minor printing, the hospital where the project occurred provided these items. Therefore, the approximate cost of this project was $348.68.

Table 1

Budget Plan

Research Expense	Number of Items	Total Cost	Reference for Cost
Childhood Trauma Questionnaire	50 questionnaires	$89.10	(Pearson, n.d.)
Data Collection Tools	5 forms	$1.10	(United Postal Service [UPS], n.d.)

Gas to and from site (3 days/week for 8 weeks)	1680 miles	$258.48	(American Automobile Association [AAA], n.d.) (Fuel Cost Calculator, n.d.) (Mapquest, n.d.)
TOTAL			**$348.68**

Timeline

The timeline for completion of the quality improvement project was seven months. The approval for the quality improvement project had already been obtained; the next phase of the project was to implement the project plan in the hospital. This happened in February of 2024. Data collection took place before the initiation of the change included in the project, mid-January 2024. Data was collected again after the change and observation phase, in March 2024. The final report, including the five-chapter write-up, was completed in August 2024.

This timeline did not include preparation for the project. When referencing preparation this included developing the project, research, project planning, obtaining approval for the project, and attending committee and staff meetings. In addition, the timeline did not include preparing the nursing education.

Protection of Human Subjects

The researcher obtained no protected health information (PHI) to report the results of this project. The patients filled out the questionnaire, but their responses were not what was being studied. What was being studied is whether or not doing this will impact providing Trauma-informed care to the patients, measured by the identification of patient trauma history and the communication of that trauma history amongst nurses.

All data collected by the student and reported to staff, other students, and faculty was assigned a number. For both areas of data collection, how many should have been done and how many were, is what was being collected. There was no PHI needed for this.

Auditing of charts was required to gather pre-intervention information and to ensure that the CTQ was being completed and then reported on the communication sheet appropriately; only numbers were collected. Therefore, PHI was not removed from the facility for any reason.

Conclusion

As stated previously, this project was important in determining whether utilizing the CTQ increased the number of patients who had their trauma history assessed and whether it increased communication of positive trauma history. This project was a quality improvement project that required no PHI. This aided in ensuring patient privacy and protection. The short timeline and the small budget required enabled implementation and allowed for inciteful results in a timely manner.

FOUR:

Findings

THE PURPOSE OF THE scholarly project was to determine if utilizing the childhood trauma questionnaire on inpatients in a behavioral health unit would improve the implementation of Trauma-informed care. The project obtained qualitative data before the project period and post-implementation. Data collection was done first by a retrospective chart review to determine the occurrence of trauma identification as well as the communication of trauma history. This chapter will discuss the evaluation methods, data analysis, and the project's findings in more detail.

Methods of Evaluation

The Childhood Trauma Questionnaire (CTQ) was distributed during the project's intervention phase. After the intervention, data collection regarding trauma identification and communication of these findings was obtained. All pre- and post-data collection was done through document/chart review and recorded on a spreadsheet. Trauma-informed care includes identifying trauma and communicating it to each other. This allowed staff to individualize the care that they provide. This project compares pre- and post-data in each of these different areas.

Quantitative Methods

To start the project, data collection was done eight weeks before the intervention. All patients newly admitted during this time frame, per a census list provided by the unit director, were selected. All these patients had their medical records reviewed, and those not meeting the inclusion criteria were excluded. The remaining patients then had their records reviewed for reports of trauma. Finally, the patients who did report trauma were compared to the communication logs during the eight-week period to determine if their report of trauma was communicated.

After the pre-intervention data collection was completed, all nurses were educated on the intervention and the project. They then carried out the intervention for eight weeks. At the end of the intervention the data collection began again. The only difference in the data collection post-intervention was that instead of the patients who met the criteria having a chart review on their report of trauma, they had their CTQs reviewed.

Setting

The setting of this project was the Behavioral Health Unit (BHU) at a local hospital. This unit is a 40-bed inpatient hospital unit that admits patients who are experiencing a mental health crisis or are in withdrawal from a substance, typically alcohol. Childhood trauma has a positive correlation to future mental health issues and substance use (Cay et al., 2022; Heany et al., 2017). Due to this, it is important that Trauma-informed care is provided to patients with those issues.

There are assigned staff who were hired to work on this unit. Since the unit is specialized in mental health and substance use, as opposed to the general medical demands of the rest of the hospital, it is uncommon for nurses to be sent to this unit to work. Part of the exclusion criteria for the study is that patients being cared for by nurses who were not hired to work on the unit must be excluded. Therefore, it is desirable to the study that the majority of the nurses working on the unit were hired to be there.

Sample

This project's purpose was to enable nurses to better provide Trauma-informed care by the identification and communication of childhood trauma in patients. This setting was, therefore, a match to the goal of the project. In addition, a higher sample size was preferred, to determine the applicability of the project on a wider scale. Since the chosen setting is a 40- bed hospital unit, there are many patients admitted to the unit, increasing the odds of having a larger sample size. In addition, the average length of stay was three to five days, allowing for a higher patient turnover and, therefore, a larger sample size.

Structure of Intervention

The steps of the intervention were to collect pre-intervention data, educate the nurses on the project and what to do, test the process for 1 week, make changes as needed for one week, then allow for the eight-week intervention period. After the eight-week intervention period post-intervention data was collected.

While this sounds simple, the expectations of the nurses were high. The nurse's role was to provide the CTQ to patients on admission to the unit, explain to them that they need to fill out the CTQ independently, and then collect it within 24 hours. After collection, the nurses were to score the questionnaire, place the results on their shift-to-shift communication log, and place the CTQ in the director of nursing's box for collection and storage.

During the two-week period of testing the intervention and making changes, it was determined that the scoring of the CTQ was to be shifted to the unit secretaries. The unit secretaries would then place the scores on the communication sheet. The secretaries also placed the CTQ in the director's box. This change was made to take some of the time-consuming burden off the nursing staff.

Data Quality and Adequacy

Many methods were utilized to ensure the quality and adequacy of the data collected. All behavioral health unit nurses, including the manager and director, were trained on the project, data collection, and the importance of accurate and complete data. In addition, the staff was responsible for carrying out the change intervention and providing all CTQ and communication logs to the director for storage.

Upon completion of the project, the researcher was the sole data collector. The researcher audited charts twice to ensure inclusion/exclusion criteria were met. The CTQ was then compared to the communication logs twice. Finally, all data that was recorded was reviewed and checked twice. Checking everything twice ensured that the data collected was accurate and that nothing was missed.

Ethical Considerations

This project had multiple ethical considerations, some that applied and others that did not. One was the involvement of live, vulnerable patients. This particular consideration did not apply to the project, as the project was a quality improvement project. The patients had the choice to participate or not. In addition, there was no testing on the patients, and what the individual patient recorded on the CTQ was not being studied, only that it was completed.

This project went through the investigational review boards (IRB) at the school and the hospital. Both boards ruled that the project was exempt from needing official IRB approval as it was a quality improvement project. In addition, the project proposal went before the hospital research committee and obtained permission to perform the project at the selected location.

Another ethical consideration was the privacy of protected health information (PHI). The researcher mitigated this by not removing any PHI from the hospital unit. All data reviews, collection, and analyses were performed on the unit. Data collection was done by obtaining a checklist of yes and no on whether different aspects of the project were completed. No patient-identifying information was needed.

Conflict of Interest

The researcher for this project was a previous employee of the organization where the study was completed. In addition, the researcher was a current student performing their practicum hours at the same organization. However, the researcher was never an official employee of the unit where the research was being conducted and did not do practicum hours on the unit where the research was being conducted.

Data Analysis and Presentation of Data

The use of the CTQ and the communication of results were the subjects of this project. The nurses at the BHU were responsible for changing their practice to utilize the CTQ and report positive trauma. The patients were responsible for filling out the CTQ truthfully and completely.

To be included in the project, the nurses who admitted the patients had to work for the BHU, not elsewhere in the hospital. This excluded any nurse sent to the unit from another unit to help. This was because these nurses were not trained at the BHU and, therefore, may not be aware of the project or the importance of it.

The patients also had criteria to be included in the project. Any patient who could not read English was not included because the CTQ had to be given to the patients to fill out the CTQ independently, and it was only available in English. Patients also had to be alert and oriented times four (to person, place, time, and situation). Some patients who are admitted are under the influence or in a psychosis. These patients may not have been able to report their childhood trauma accurately.

Descriptive Statistics

The BHU is an inpatient hospital unit that admits patients who are experiencing a mental health crisis or are in withdrawal from a substance. The patients that are admitted to this unit, during the time of the project, were mixed gender and race, though they were predominantly white females. The admission age is 18 years old and over; however, most patients admitted during the time of the project fell between 25 and 65. No patients were excluded due to their race, gender, or age.

Variability

The pre-intervention and post-intervention data reviews were done over the same period of time, eight weeks. This allowed for some consistency in the results. Another factor that allowed for consistency was following the inclusion and exclusion criteria for the entire project. The unit the project was done on has a high turnover rate, which allowed for a larger sample size, making the pre- and post-intervention data more significant.

Despite the areas of consistency, there were still some expected variances. The exact number of patients is one variance. The number of admissions to the BHU was not likely to be the same. As with any area in healthcare, one cannot control how many patients are getting admitted. Another expected variance is the inclusion and exclusion criteria affecting the population size, considering that some patients refused to take the CTQ.

Other variances included the nurses. Not every nurse was consistent in providing the CTQ to the patients, as well as collecting them; not every secretary was consistent about reporting results to the communication sheets. In other words, compliance with the project varied.

Despite the expected variances, it was the expectation that there was an increase in attempting to identify a patient's trauma history. It was expected that there would be an increase in the communication of positive trauma history. While the project sizes varied, the Z-Test being used for data analysis accounted for the differences and was able to determine if the data was significant, regardless of the different sizes.

Results

In discussing the results of this project, it was important to reflect on many areas, not just the outcome. These areas of reflection included the process, associations, and unintended consequences. By reflecting on all of the areas, the project's results can be more fully understood and appreciated.

Outcomes of Intervention

Upon data collection and review, it was determined that the number of patients who were identified as having a history of trauma did not have a statistically significant increase post-intervention than the patients before the intervention, $z = 8.14$ $p = 1.00$. (See Table 2).

In the pre-intervention data collection, trauma history was inquired about in 223 patients out of the 225 selected for the project. This equates to 95% of the patients. Post-intervention, this percentage decreased. Only 86 patients out of 139 completed the CTQ.

This means that only 62% had trauma history inquired about; see Figure 1.

Patients had their trauma history communicated statistically significantly more of the time after the intervention than patients before the intervention, z= 8.93 and p= .00, (See Table 3). In the pre-intervention data collection, trauma history was communicated in 21 out of the 86 patients identified with trauma. This equates to 24% of the patients. Post-intervention, this percentage increased. 61 out of 62, or 98% of patients, had their trauma history communicated; see Figure 2.

While having a decrease in asking patients about their trauma was not what was hypothesized, there are multiple possible reasons for this outcome. Possible reasons for this outcome include the smaller sample size and some nurses not providing the CTQ to their patients. However, despite the decrease in trauma history being asked about, the information obtained was much more detailed. Before the CTQ, patients were only generally asked if they had a history of trauma. However, with the CTQ, the trauma was able to be broken down into severity levels of different types of traumas: emotional abuse, physical abuse, sexual abuse, emotional neglect, and physical neglect.

Despite the results of the first measure, trauma identification, the second measure of improving the communication of positive trauma results was highly successful. Pre-intervention data showed that only 21 patients out of the 86 that trauma was identified had their trauma history communicated to the between-shift communication logs. This means that trauma history was only communicated from shift to shift on 24% of the patients that it should have been. However, post-intervention trauma history was communicated on 61 out of 62 patients. This means it was communicated on 98% of the patients, see Figure 2.

Table 2

Identification of Childhood Trauma

	Trauma Identified	Sample Size	P-Level
Pre- Intervention	223 (94.98%)	225	1.00
Post-Intervention	86 (61.87%)	139	

Note. Confidence interval 95% with lower limit of -.4157 and upper limit of -.2447.

Figure 1

Identification of Childhood Trauma

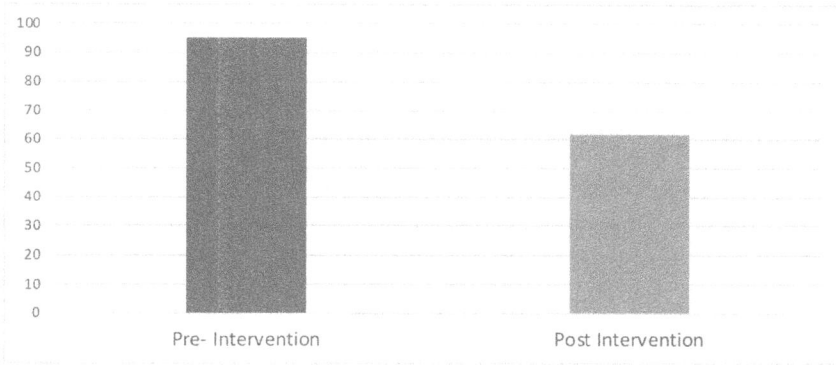

Note. Measure number one.

Table 3

Communication of Trauma History

Trauma Communicated		Sample Size	P-Level
Pre- Intervention	21 (24.42%)	86	0.00
Post-Intervention	61 (98.39%)	62	

Note. Confidence interval 95% with lower limit of .6436 and lower limit of .8357.

Figure 2

Communication of Trauma History

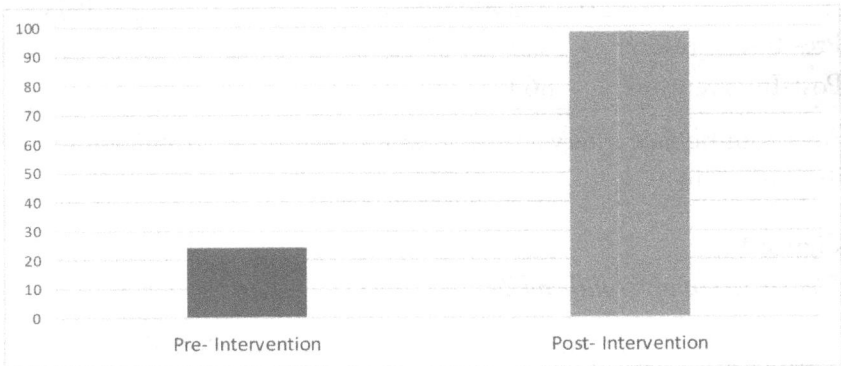

Note. Measure number two.

Facilitators and Barriers

There were multiple associations between interventions and outcomes for this project. These associations included both facilitators and barriers. Some of the identified facilitators of this project, as well as interventions and outcomes, doubled as a barrier.

One facilitator was that the nurses, director of nursing, and nursing manager were all educated on the project. The goal for educating the nurses was 100%, which was achieved. Another facilitator was that the staff had a lot of positive feedback regarding education. This was considered a facilitator because if the staff were not engaged in the project, they would be unlikely to do their part in its success. The last facilitator, the director of nursing, chose the topic on which research was going to be conducted. She wanted research to focus on improving Trauma-informed care. Her support from day one assisted the researcher in obtaining staff support and access to records.

The first barrier was that although the director chose the topic to be studied, there was little leadership enforcement and staff accountability. Due to this, a couple of nurses did not follow through with providing the CTQ to patients that they admitted, despite the education they received. Another barrier was the smaller sample size during the post-intervention data collection period. Multiple things affected the post-intervention sample size, including losing week eight data, fewer admissions, nurses not offering the CTQ, and more float staff (which led increased exclusion).

The final barrier identified was that the secretaries were uneducated on the project and intervention. They were not educated because, originally, the nurses were to perform all aspects of the CTQ process. However, this was deemed to be too time-consuming. Therefore, the scoring, reporting, and collecting of the CTQ were moved to the secretaries during the intervention period.

Unintended Consequences

There were quite a few unintended consequences of the project. These consequences include both beneficial outcomes and unexpected failures. An unexpected failure of this project was that trauma history was not assessed in more patients than before the intervention. Before the intervention, trauma history was assessed 94.89% of the time. However, post-intervention, trauma history was assessed by the CTQ, only 61.87% of the time. This could be attributed to the nursing staff not providing the CTQ and patients refusing to participate in filling it out.

In contrast, an unexpected benefit was that the history of trauma, despite it not being asked about as frequently, was more accurately identified. It was determined that before utilizing the CTQ, patients denied having a trauma history on admission when they later disclosed that they did, 15.32% of the time. Post implementation of the CTQ, it was determined that this false reporting dropped to 3.47%. This is an improvement in accurately identifying childhood trauma by 11.85%.

Figure 3

Adults with Trauma

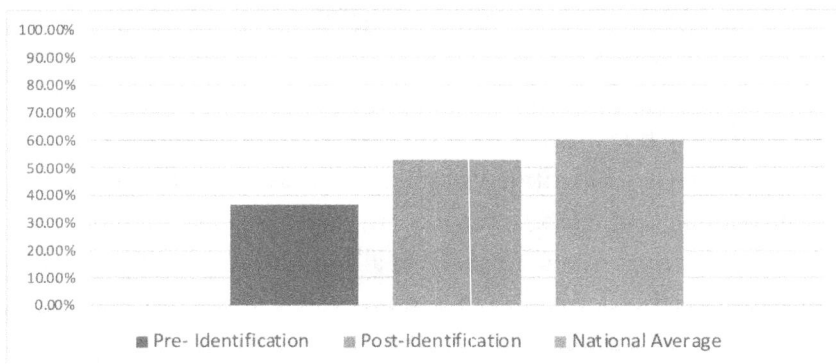

Note. Comparison of project data to the national average.

Another benefit was that even though the CTQ was not completed as much as the pre-intervention way of identifying trauma, trauma was identified in more patients (See Figure 3). This speaks to the efficacy of the CTQ, and potentially the education, over the previous screening tool being utilized. Prior to this project, 36.6% of patients reported having a trauma history. However, post intervention, this number increased to 53.06%, which is closer to the national average of approximately 60% (Swedo et al., 2023).

Conclusion

While the project measures did not necessarily come out as expected, it was still considered successful. Though it was discovered that the CTQ might potentially decrease the number of times patients are asked about their trauma history when used, the CTQ was found to be more sensitive in identifying childhood trauma and provides significantly more information about the type of trauma the patient has experienced.

The intervention was also shown to significantly increase the communication of patient trauma amongst staff from shift to shift.

This is important because Trauma-informed care cannot be provided if the staff does not know about the patient's trauma history. The improved details received from the CTQ also allow the care to be further individualized to each patient. A more in-depth discussion of these results will follow in chapter 5.

FIVE:

Discussion

THIS PROJECT HAS HIGHLIGHTED the importance of reliable and valid screening tools in identifying childhood trauma. The Childhood Trauma Questionnaire (CTQ) was this project's reliable and valid tool (Georgieva et al., 2021; Xiang et al., 2021). In improving Trauma-informed care, this project found that utilizing the CTQ improved data accuracy and increased the detail in the data received. While the CTQ itself was not being studied, it showed superiority to the general questions about whether a patient had a trauma history.

Additionally, the entire intervention improved communication among staff. Previously, the nurses would ask the patients about their trauma history on admission. This would trigger the nurse to document that the patient had trauma in the electronic health record. That was where the process stopped. To determine if a patient had a traumatic past, this information would have to be searched for. However, with this project, nearly all reports of trauma history were reported to the communication log from shift-to-shift.

Strengths

There were three main strengths to this project. The first was that the accuracy of the data obtained improved from pre- to post-intervention. The second was that the communication of patient trauma history increased from pre- to post-intervention. Finally, the amount of detail obtained regarding a patient's trauma history also improved.

Data accuracy improved, as illustrated in Chapter 4: Data Analysis. Before the intervention, it was identified that 15.32% of patients denied having a trauma history on admission and later reported that they did. Post-intervention, this number decreased to 3.47%. This shows that, after utilizing the CTQ, patients were more likely to disclose their trauma history the first time. This was a significant finding, because without accurate disclosure, Trauma-informed care cannot be provided when it may be needed. The CTQ asking more in-depth questions, and the patients being expected to fill out on their own, in privacy, may have attributed to this improvement.

An important aspect of Trauma-informed care is identifying patients who have experienced trauma. However, identification means nothing if this information is not shared, so that nurses can tailor their care to each patient's specific needs. Before this project, communication of a patient's trauma history was only happening 24% of the time. However, post-intervention increased to 98%. This increase could be attributed to the increased focus placed on trauma identification and Trauma-informed care. It could also be attributed to the nurses being educated on the project itself, the importance of communication in Trauma-informed care, and the expectations that trauma history be communicated. Regardless of the reason, this improvement was significant.

Before this project, when assessing trauma history, patients were asked to positively or negatively identify if they had a history of trauma. This was a yes or no question. However, when utilizing the

CTQ, patients answered a series of questions regarding their childhood. These questions were then broken down into different types of traumas: emotional abuse, physical abuse, sexual abuse, emotional neglect, and physical neglect. Each type of trauma was then able to be assigned a severity level. This severity level was reported to the communication logs that the staff used to do an end-of-shift report to the next shift. Having more information assisted the nurses and other healthcare workers in tailoring the care that they provided to each individual patient's needs.

Nursing and leadership involvement and support in this project assisted in the success of the project. Much of the project relied on the staff utilizing the CTQ, explaining it to patients, collecting, scoring, and reporting the results. None of this would have been accomplished without their support for the project.

Limitations

As with any study or project, some limitations can still be identified despite the strengths. One such limitation was nurse compliance. While most nurses complied with the project expectations, such as handing out the CTQ to patients on admission, there was a margin of error where this was not completed. To mitigate this risk, there was a trial period where the intervention was started but was not included in the eight-week project period. This allowed the researcher to assess compliance and follow up with staff that were not meeting expectations. Unfortunately, there were still some situations where the nurses did not provide the CTQ.

Another limitation was leadership involvement, or lack thereof, in enforcing the process and expectations. To mitigate this risk, the leaders of the unit played a huge role in determining the project topic. In addition, they were kept up to date on the project plans, timeline, and results. Each portion of the project met their approval before continuing to the next steps. However, despite these measures, the leadership team remained "hands-off" with educating, following up, and holding staff accountable to the expectations of the project and quality improvement changes. In addition, there were many steps in the change process, which offered more room for error, and non-compliance.

The project sizes, pre- and post-intervention, varied as well. This results from lower admission rates during the intervention data period, more patients refusing the CTQ, and missing data. Admission rates to a hospital unit are not something that could be controlled. However, education was done on the CTQ and how nurses should have provided it to patients. This included education on the nurses explaining the importance of the CTQ to patients so that they understood the need to fill it out.

Unfortunately, there was a higher rate of refusal with the CTQ than with the yes or no questions previously asked about trauma history. In addition, as referenced in Chapter 4: Data Analysis, there was a week's worth of missing data from the intervention period. While data collection and storage were planned for and discussed in-depth, the unit director could not locate the last week, week 8 of the intervention period.

Missing Data

A disclosure needs to be made regarding missing data in this project. The pre-intervention data includes eight weeks of information. However, the post-intervention data only includes seven weeks. As part of the project, the unit secretaries were to give the completed CTQs to the unit director, who was to store them for the researcher. Unfortunately, upon retrieval of the CTQs for data collection, it was discovered that week eight of the intervention period was not accounted for. Due to this, the post-intervention data is incomplete and week eight could not be included in the evaluation and analysis of the results. This drastically affected the post-intervention sample size.

Post-Implementation Insights

Post-implementation, there were a few insights gleaned from the process. One such insight was that the entire staff should have been educated on the project and process. Originally, it was decided that the nursing staff would own the process changes. However, it was determined during the project that the process was too lengthy and had too many steps for the nurses to own. While the steps of the project were simple, it became too time-consuming. Due to this, the scoring and reporting of the results was shifted to the secretaries. While the secretaries fully supported the project and changes to their routine, they never received the original education on the project, its importance, and expectations.

Accountability was another insight. While most of the nurses and secretaries followed the expectations of the project, some did not. Accountability was a barrier to the project but could have been a facilitator. In this scenario, leadership accountability of themselves as well as staff would have been useful. With increased accountability, the sample sizes may have been more similar. This could have decreased the patient refusals, decreased the number of times nurses did not provide the CTQ, and assisted in the appropriate maintenance of data so that it was not lost.

Interpretation

There were two expected outcomes of this project. The first was that the CTQ would be used to assess trauma history more frequently than the previous method being utilized. This was found not to be the case. Reasons for this include the staff compliance with administering the questionnaire, as well as patient refusal to utilize the questionnaire. It was found that refusal to utilize the questionnaire increased, compared to the previous method. This could have been due to the lengthy questionnaire and some patients not wanting to disclose such personal information. In addition, the patients were expected to complete the questionnaire independently, as opposed to the nurses asking the questions.

The second expected outcome was that when trauma history was identified, it would be communicated more often than it was before the intervention. This was found to be true. Reasons for this include the higher focus on Trauma-informed care, training provided to all nurses, and the project itself. The nurses were trained on the project and the importance of identifying and communicating trauma.

Implications for Future Research

One recommendation for additional research is having the staff members ask the CTQ questions as part of their assessment, instead of the patients being asked to fill it out. This would help to determine whether the patient filling it out privately led to the increase in accurate responses, or whether it was in-depth questions.

Another recommendation is to have the social workers administer the questionnaire. This would help to determine if there is a difference between social workers versus nurses doing this. Would the social workers be more compliant? Would more patients fill it out?

Finally, trying other questionnaires within this same project format is another recommendation. This will show whether other questionnaires are just as effective, or if it was because the CTQ specifically was chosen. There is a question as to whether shorter less invasive questionnaires could increase the number of patients willing to fill it out without compromising the accuracy of the information obtained.

Implications for Future Practice

Implications to practice for this research include identifying childhood trauma and improving communication amongst staff to tailor the care that is being provided to each individual patient (Trauma-informed care). Despite the higher rate of not using the CTQ, this research showed that using a reliable, valid, and more specific tool can improve the information obtained from patients, as well as increase their admission of positive trauma history. Placing a higher focus on and adjusting work processes was also shown to increase communication amongst staff significantly.

Implications for Healthcare Policy

Health policy is essential to promote wellness and ensure that large scale health goals are met, and standards of care are upheld. Trauma-informed care, when provided effectively, has been shown to decrease the number of unplanned discharges (Hales et al., 2018). Decreasing the number of unplanned discharges will decrease readmission. This project improved the administration of Trauma-informed care. With decreased readmission rates there will be a decreased demand on the healthcare system.

Policy should include requiring identification of childhood trauma on admission of patients to the hospital and then individualization of their treatment plans/ plan of care, based on these findings. This will leave it open to how childhood trauma is identified. It will also allow organizations to utilize the most appropriate tool for their clientele. The importance should be placed on efficiently identifying childhood trauma, not on the tool used.

Recommendations and Conclusions

Based on the findings of this project, it was concluded that using the CTQ improves the accuracy and specificity of reported trauma. It was also concluded that communication about reported trauma can be improved. Both are aspects of Trauma-informed care; therefore, it is reasonable to say that utilizing the CTQ and improving communication does improve Trauma-informed care.

Considerations for the sustainability of this project were also discussed with the unit director and manager. One consideration was using the current two-question identification process as a backup for patients who refuse the CTQ. While this process was not shown to be as sensitive and accurate, some information could be considered better than none.

Another consideration was creating a process to scan the CTQ into the patient's chart. This would not only allow for the information to be maintained as part of their medical record but also decrease the likelihood of misplacing the questionnaires. This was especially important due to the director's history of not retaining the documents.

Finally, ensuring higher accountability of staff and leaders is essential. For this project, despite engaging leadership and performing the project on a topic that they chose, there was little leadership involvement and support. This project has been shown to be successful, but without the leaders holding the staff accountable for the changes, it is unlikely to continue to succeed.

Plan for Sustainability

The plan for sustainability of this project and change comes with action and considerations for the unit and hospital it was done at. The first action to be taken was to review the results, strengths, limitations, and recommendations with the hospital research committee, director of nursing, and manager of nursing. To continue this change within the organization, it is imperative that everyone understand the results and the implications of the findings.

The next action was to supply those same individuals and committees with contact information to obtain permission to replicate the CTQ within the hospital. Permission was previously obtained for the CTQ to be used for this project, but it was only replicable for the purpose of the project itself. Further use would require purchasing the CTQ or obtaining permission to replicate it.

Plan for Dissemination

The plan for dissemination of this project is not linear. Instead, it is more of a broad outline of tasks. First is word of mouth. This includes talking about the project and the successful changes made on the unit. The hospital where the project was completed is part of a larger organization. Due to this, meeting with the aforementioned committees will allow for the project to be disseminated on a larger scale.

Another part of dissemination is publication. This five-chapter report will be shortened and summarized to include all key points, data, and outcomes. It will then be sent to multiple journals and magazines to be peer-reviewed and eventually published. By doing this, the word will spread, and hopefully, there will be more research to follow.

The final piece to disseminate the findings of this project is spreading the information via conferences. The more people hear about the importance of identifying and communicating childhood trauma, the more Trauma-informed care can be utilized. Posters and infographics will be created for presentation and dissemination.

Conclusion

Healthcare has come a long way in the last century, especially around mental health. It is now generally accepted that trauma can impact all aspects of our lives. However, despite knowing this, Trauma-informed care is a newer concept. The focus now needs to be on how to provide it adequately. This starts with the identification and communication of trauma.

References

Aloba, O., Opakunle, T., & Ogunrinu, O. (2020). Childhood trauma questionnaire-short form (CTQ-SF): Dimensionality, validity, reliability, and gender invariance among Nigerian adolescents. *Child Abuse and Neglect, 101*. https://doi.org/10.1016/j.chiabu.2020.104357

American Automobile Association (AAA) (n.d.). *Gas prices*. Retrieved on October 21, 2023, from https://gasprices.aaa.com/?state=KS

American Psychiatric Association. (2021). *What is somatic symptom disorder?* Psychiatry.org. Retrieved from https://www.psychiatry.org/patients-families/somatic-symptom-disorder/what-is-somatic-symptom-disorder#:~:text=Somatic%20symptom%20disorder%20is%20diagnosed,relating%20to%20the%20physical%20symptoms.

Angelakis, I., Gillespie, E. L., & Panagioti, M. (2019). Childhood maltreatment and adult suicidality: A comprehensive systematic review with meta-analysis. *Psychological Medicine, 49*(07), 1057–1078. https://doi.org/10.1017/s0033291718003823

Behr Gomes Jardim, G., Novelo, M., Spanemberg, L., von Gunten, A., Engroff, P., Nogueira, E. L., & Cataldo Neto, A. (2018). Influence of childhood abuse and neglect subtypes on late-life suicide risk beyond depression. *Child Abuse & Neglect, 80*, 249–256. https://doi.org/10.1016/j.chiabu.2018.03.029

Bloomfield, M. A., Yusuf, F. N., Srinivasan, R., Kelleher, I., Bell, V., & Pitman, A. (2020). Trauma-informed care for adult survivors of developmental trauma with psychotic and dissociative symptoms: A systematic review of Intervention Studies. *The Lancet Psychiatry, 7*(5), 449–462. https://doi.org/10.1016/s2215-0366(20)30041-9

Caruth, C. (1995). *Trauma: Explorations in memory.* Johns Hopkins Univ. Press.

Cay, M., Chouinard, V.-A., Hall, M.-H., & Shinn, A. K. (2022). Test-retest reliability of the Childhood Trauma Questionnaire in psychotic disorders. *Journal of Psychiatric Research, 156*, 78–83. https://doi.org/10.1016/j.jpsychires.2022.09.053

Center for Healthcare Strategy. (2022, July 7). *What is Trauma-informed care?* Trauma-informed Care Implementation Resource Center. Retrieved from https://www.traumainformed-care.chcs.org/what-is-Trauma-informed-care/

Cilia Vincenti, S., Grech, P., & Scerri, J. (2021). Psychiatric hospital nurses' attitudes towards trauma-informed care. *Journal of Psychiatric and Mental Health Nursing, 29*(1), 75–85. https://doi.org/10.1111/jpm.12747

Copeland, W. E., Shanahan, L., Hinesley, J., Chan, R. F., Aberg, K. A., Fairbank, J. A., van den Oord, E. J., & Costello, E. J. (2018). Association of childhood trauma exposure with adult psychiatric disorders and functional outcomes. *JAMA Network Open, 1*(7). https://doi.org/10.1001/jamanet-workopen.2018.4493

Dalton, M., Harrison, J., Malin, A., & Leavey, C. (2018). Factors that influence nurses' assessment of patient acuity and response to acute deterioration. *British Journal of Nursing, 27*(4), 212–218. https://doi.org/10.12968/bjon.2018.27.4.212

Fuel Cost Calculator (n.d.). *Fuel cost.* Retrieved on October 21, 2023, from https://www.calculator.net/fuel-cost-calculator.html?tripdistance=70&tripdistanceunit=miles&fuelefficiency=22&fuelefficiencyunit=mpg&gasprice=3.386&gaspriceunit=gallon&x=77&y=23

Gawęda, Ł., Pionke, R., Krężołek, M., Frydecka, D., Nelson, B., & Cechnicki, A. (2019). The interplay between childhood trauma, cognitive biases, psychotic-like experiences and depression and their additive impact on predicting lifetime suicidal behavior in young adults. *Psychological Medicine, 50*(1), 116–124. https://doi.org/10.1017/s0033291718004026

Georgieva, S., Tomas, J. M., & Navarro-Pérez, J. J. (2021). Systematic review and critical appraisal of Childhood Trauma Questionnaire — short form (CTQ-SF). *Child Abuse & Neglect, 120*, 105223. https://doi.org/10.1016/j.chiabu.2021.105223

Grattan, R. E., Lara, N., Botello, R. M., Tryon, V. L., Maguire, A. M., Carter, C. S., & Niendam, T. A. (2019). A history of trauma is associated with aggression, depression, non-suicidal self-injury behavior, and suicide ideation in first-episode psychosis. *Journal of Clinical Medicine, 8*(7), 1082. https://doi.org/10.3390/jcm8071082

Hagborg, J. M., Kalin, T., & Gerdner, A. (2022). The Childhood Trauma Questionnaire—short form (CTQ-SF) used with adolescents – methodological report from clinical and community samples. *Journal of Child & Adolescent Trauma, 15*(4), 1199–1213. https://doi.org/10.1007/s40653-022-00443-8

Hales, T. W., Green, S. A., Bissonette, S., Warden, A., Diebold, J., Koury, S. P., & Nochajski, T. H. (2018). Trauma-informed care outcome study. *Research on Social Work Practice, 29*(5), 529–539. https://doi.org/10.1177/1049731518766618

Heany, S. J., Groenewold, N. A., Uhlmann, A., Dalvie, S., Stein, D. J., & Brooks, S. J. (2017). The neural correlates of childhood trauma questionnaire scores in adults: A meta-analysis and review of Functional Magnetic Resonance Imaging Studies. *Development and Psychopathology, 30*(4), 1475–1485. https://doi.org/10.1017/s0954579417001717

Isobel, S., Gladstone, B., Goodyear, M., Furness, T., & Foster, K. (2020). A qualitative inquiry into psychiatrists' perspectives on the relationship of psychological trauma to mental illness and treatment: Implications for Trauma-informed care. *Journal of Mental Health, 30*(6), 667–673. https://doi.org/10.1080/09638237.2020.1714012

Korchmaros, J. D., Greene, A., & Murphy, S. (2020). Implementing Trauma-informed research-supported treatment: Fidelity, feasibility, and acceptability. *Child and Adolescent Social Work*

Journal, 38(1), 101–113. https://doi.org/10.1007/s10560-020-00671-7

Kramer, M. K., & Chinn, P. L. (2013). *Integrated theory and knowledge development in nursing* (8th ed.). Elsevier.

Kratzer, L., Knefel, M., Haselgruber, A., Heinz, P., Schennach, R., & Karatzias, T. (2021). Co-occurrence of severe PTSD, somatic symptoms and dissociation in a large sample of childhood trauma inpatients: A network analysis. *European Archives of Psychiatry and Clinical Neuroscience, 272*(5), 897–908. https://doi.org/10.1007/s00406-021-01342-z

Mambrol, N. (2020, July 15). *Trauma studies.* Literary Theory and Criticism. https://literariness.org/2018/12/19/trauma-studies/#:~:text=In%20the%20traditional%20trauma%20model,experience%20irrevocably%20damages%20the%20psyche.

Mapquest (n.d.). *Mileage.* Retrieved on October 21, 2023, from https://www.mapquest.com/directions/from/us/ks/baldwin-city/66006-7007/509-heritage-dr-38.77728,-95.16854/to/us/kansas/adventhealth-shawnee-mission-425393360

Mayo Foundation for Medical Education and Research. (2022, December 13). *Dissociative disorders.* Mayo Clinic. https://www.mayoclinic.org/diseases-conditions/dissociative-disorders/symptoms-causes/syc-20355215

Northwestern University. (2020, June 22). *What is child trauma?* Center for Child Trauma Assessment and Service Planning. Retrieved from https://cctasi.northwestern.edu/child-trauma/

Oquendo, M. A., Galfalvy, H. C., Choo, T.-H., Kandlur, R., Burke, A. K., Sublette, M. E., Miller, J. M., Mann, J. J., & Stanley, B. H. (2020). Highly variable suicidal ideation: A phenotypic marker for stress induced suicide risk. *Molecular Psychiatry, 26*(9), 5079–5086. https://doi.org/10.1038/s41380-020-0819-0

Ozakar Akca, S., Oztas, G., Karadere, M. E., & Yazla Asafov, E. (2021). Childhood trauma and its relationship with suicide probability and self-esteem: A case study in a university in Turkey. *Perspectives in Psychiatric Care, 58*(4), 1839–1846. https://doi.org/10.1111/ppc.12997

Pearson (n.d.). Childhood trauma questionnaire: A retrospective self-report. Retrieved on October 21, 2023 from https://www.pearsonassessments.com/store/usassessments/en/Store/Professional-Assessments/Personality-%26-Biopsychosocial/Childhood-Trauma-Questionnaire%3A-A-Retrospective-Self-Report/p/100000446.html

Polit, D. F., & Beck, C. T. (2021). *Nursing research generating and assessing evidence for nursing practice* (11th Ed.). Wolters Kluwer.

Ranjbar, N., Erb, M., Mohammad, O., & Moreno, F. A. (2020). Trauma-informed care and cultural humility in the mental health care of people from Minoritized Communities. *Focus, 18*(1), 8–15. https://doi.org/10.1176/appi.focus.20190027

Schmidt, M. R., Narayan, A. J., Atzl, V. M., Rivera, L. M., & Lieberman, A. F. (2018). Childhood maltreatment on the Adverse Childhood Experiences (ACES) scale versus The Childhood Trauma Questionnaire (CTQ) in a perinatal sample. *Journal of Aggression, Maltreatment & Trauma, 29*(1), 38–56. https://doi.org/10.1080/10926771.2018.1524806

Substance Abuse and Mental Health Services Association [SAMH-SA]. (2022, September). *Understanding child trauma.* SAM-HSA. October 21, 2022, from https://www.samhsa.gov/child-trauma/understanding-child-trauma

Swedo, E. A., Aslam, M. V., Dahlberg, L. L., Niolon, P. H., Guinn, A. S., Simon, T. R., & Mercy, J. A. (2023). Prevalence of adverse childhood experiences among U.S. adults — behavioral risk factor surveillance system, 2011–2020. *MMWR. Morbidity and Mortality Weekly Report, 72*(26), 707–715. https://doi.org/10.15585/mmwr.mm7226a2

United Postal Service (UPS) (n.d.). *Printing services.* Retrieved on October 21,2023 from, https://locations.theupsstore.com/ks/lawrence/2040-w-31st-st/all-printing-services.

Viscusi, W. K. (2020). Extending the domain of the value of a statistical life. *Journal of Benefit-Cost Analysis, 12*(1), 1–23. https://doi.org/10.1017/bca.2020.19

Wakefield, M. K., Williams, D. R., Menestrel, S. L., & Flaubert, J. L. (2021). *The Future of Nursing 2020-2030: Charting a path to achieve health equity.* The National Academies Press.

Xiang, Z., Liu, Z., Cao, H., Wu, Z., & Long, Y. (2021). Evaluation on long-term test–retest reliability of the short-form childhood trauma questionnaire in patients with schizophrenia. *Psychology Research and Behavior Management, Volume 14,* 1033–1040. https://doi.org/10.2147/prbm.s316398

www.ingramcontent.com/pod-product-compliance
Lightning Source LLC
Chambersburg PA
CBHW070759300326
41914CB00053B/733